Herbs Tha

Fatigue

Time-Tested Herbal Remedies

No Side-effects

by

Prayank

Contents

Introduction

Fatigue is usually associated with physical and/or mental weakness. Physical fatigue is the inability to continue functioning at the level of one's normal abilities. It becomes particularly noticeable during heavy exercise. Mental fatigue manifests in sleepiness.

Fatigue is a non-specific symptom, which means that it has many possible causes. Usually occupations that require an individual to work long hours or stay up overnight can lead to fatigue.

In the book, you will find brief details of herbs that can be used to overcome fatigue. It also gives you an option to choose the herb that is easily available in your locality.

Herb names may be different in different places, hence you should rely on botanical names to find how it is known in a particular place/location.

Though there are people who treat ailments inexpensively with herbal remedies, most consider it as the last minute miracle worker once all other avenues of treatments have been exhausted.

Such an approach discounts the sophisticated and elaborately documented information dealing with specific medicinal applications of herbs for specific complaints. The methods of herbal remedies are designed for optimum beneficial use and tested innumerable times in actual practice.

1. <u>Aloe</u>

(Aloe vera)

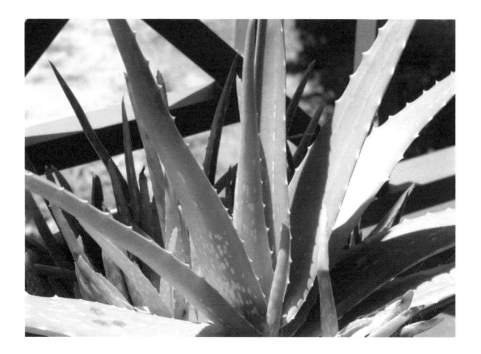

General

Aloe is a species of succulent plant that bears thorny lance-like leaves but is a favourite herb in beauty products.

The fresh juice from leaves is yellowish in colour but acquires a brownish black colour on drying. The pulp is quite bitter to taste, and emits a somewhat offensive smell. It contains the active principle aloins.

Profile

Botanical Name : Aloe vera

Other Species : Aloe barbadenesis

Family : Liliaceae

Appearance : The fibrous root produces a rosette of succulent, lance-like leaves, whitish green on both sides with spines on the margins. Flowers - orange or yellow to purplish, in racemes. Fruit - a triangular capsule, ellipsoid-oblong.

Medicinal Parts : The gel-like pulp obtained on peeling the leaves and its dried form (powder); leaves.

Distribution : Widely cultivated throughout the world.

Prescription and Dose

Take 1/10 tsp gel with a pinch of turmeric powder.

2. <u>Arkh</u>

(Calotropis gigantea)

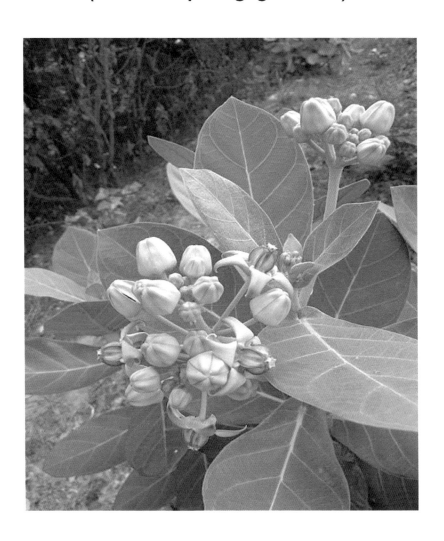

General

Although the plant is attractive to look at and medicinally useful, it gives off a foul smell. The plant blooms round the year. The plant's Sanskrit name refer to its strong, caustic action.

It is a large shrub growing to 4 m tall. It has clusters of waxy flowers that are either white or lavender in colour. Each flower consists of five pointed petals and a small, elegant "crown" rising from the center, which holds the stamens. The plant has oval, light green leaves and milky stem.

Profile

Botanical Name : Calotropis gigantea

Other Species : Calotropis procera

Family : Asclepiadoideae

Appearance : Erect pale greyish shrub covered with white cottony coat. Leaves - simple, ear shaped at base. Flowers - lilac or dull white. Fruits - in pairs, resemble mangoes, containing loose, silky and fibrous growth.

Medicinal Parts : Flowers, latex, leaves, root

Distribution : Native to Cambodia, Indonesia, Malaysia, Philippines, Thailand, Sri Lanka, India and China.

Prescription and Dose

Take some root bark and powder finely. Mix it with equal quantity of palm sugar and store.

Take one or two pinches mixed in a glass of warm milk at bedtime.

3. <u>Ashwagandha</u>
(Withania somnifera)

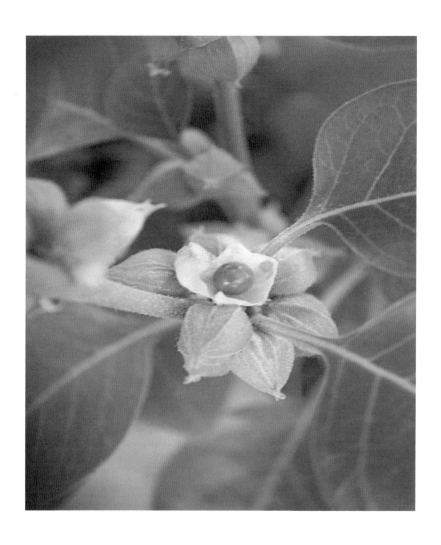

General

The Sanskrit name of the plant refers to the peculiar odour of its roots - akin to that of a stable full of horses. Ashwagandha is to Indians what ginseng is to Chinese. It grows wild in certain parts of Rajasthan in India; but most of this herb available in marketplace is from cultivated plants which are reported to differ from wild ones in their medicinal properties, though the alkaloids present are the same.

Profile

Botanical Name : Withania somnifera

Other Species : Withania ashwagandha

Family : Solanaceae

Appearance : Erect, evergreen hairy shrub. Roots - stout, fleshy, whitish brown. Leaves - simple, egg shaped. Flowers - inconspicuous, light green or pale yellow, in clusters. Fruits - berries, small, orange-red when mature, enclosed by enlarged calyx. Seeds - kidney shaped, yellow.

Medicinal Parts : Root, leaves.

Distribution : Found throughout the drier parts of India as wild shrub, and is cultivated particularly in Madhya Pradesh, Punjab and Rajasthan in India. It is also found in Nepal.

Prescription and Dose

Prepare ashwagandha root milk powder - boil the root in milk and then dry in shade. When completely dry, grind it into a very fine powder.

Take 1/2 tsp root-milk powder with 1 tsp honey or 1 cup milk twice daily.

4. <u>Bone-Setter</u>

(Cissus quadrangularis)

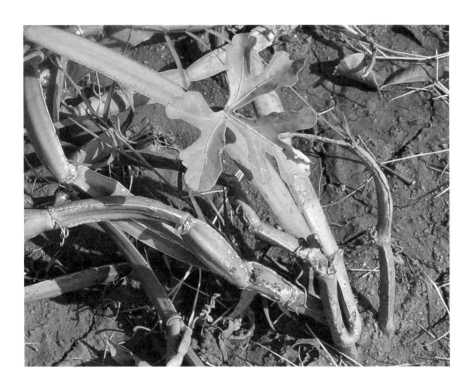

General

Bone-setter is a perennial plant of the grape family. It is commonly known as Veldt Grape or Devil's Backbone. As the name suggests, it is often used in healing broken bones. But this oddly-shaped climber is used for obesity cure too.

Profile

Botanical Name : Cissus quadrangularis

Other Species : Cissus succulenta, Vitis quadrangularis, Vitis succulenta

Family : Vitaceae

Appearance : A climber found trailing over bushes. Stem - 4-angular, fleshy and thick. Leaves - oval, found at nodes opposite a tendril. Flowers - small, in bunches, petals greenish yellow with red tips.

Medicinal Parts : The whole plant.

Distribution : Found in drier parts of Indian peninsula, Africa, Arabia and Southeast Asia. It has been imported to Brazil and the southern United States.

Prescription and Dose

Prepare ash of bone-setter: Crush the plant thoroughly and mix it with common salt (3:1 ratio). Place this mixture in a clay bowl. Seal the bowl mouth with another clay pot using - wheat flour paste or earth clay. The bowl is then fired in a kiln. When firing is complete, open the bowl mouth. You should get gray coloured ash - remnants of bone-setter. Store this ash in a bottle for use.

Take a pinch of the ash along with a pinch of nutmeg. Mix the powders with 1 tsp ghee and eat 3 times a day for a week.

5. <u>Brahmi</u>

(Bacopa monnieri)

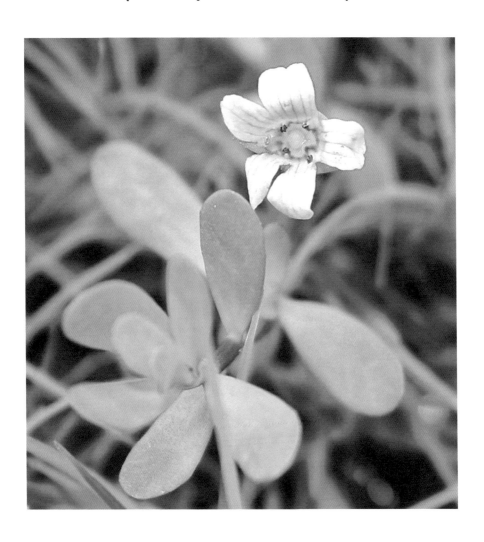

General

Brahmi is also the name given to mandukparni (Centella asiatica), particularly in north India but they are different herbs.

A perennial, creeping herb whose habitat includes wetlands and muddy shores. This herb is usually used for nervous disorders such as insanity, epilepsy, neurasthenia, nervous breakdown etc. The plant contains an alkaloid, related to strychnine, but less toxic and hence capable of safe use by those who want to stimulate the intellect and the faculty of speech. It is also used to strengthen and tone the heart muscles.

Profile

Botanical Name : Bacopa monnieri

Other Species : Herpestis monnieria, Monnieri cuneifolia, Lysimachia monnieri

Family : Fabaceae

Sub-family : Scrophlariaceae

Appearance : A small, prostrate herb with ascending branches. Roots arise on the nodes of stem. Leaves - fleshy, oblong with obscure veins. Flowers - bluish white or lilac. Fruit - egg like with persistent style.

Medicinal Parts : Leaves, fruits, the whole plant

Distribution: It commonly grows in marshy areas throughout India, Nepal, Sri Lanka, China, Taiwan, and Vietnam, and is also found in Florida, Hawaii and other southern states of the USA where it can be grown in damp conditions by the pond or bog garden.

Prescription and Dose

Boil 1 teacup fresh juice of the plant along with 1 teacup ghee. Take 1 tsp twice a day for a few days.

6. Coriander

(Coriandrum sativum)

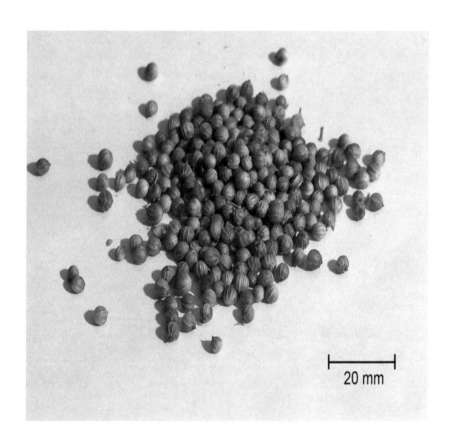

20 mm

General

Coriander (Coriandrum sativum), also known as cilantro, Chinese parsley or dhania is an annual herb, well known for its carminative and cooling properties. Both leaves of coriander and its seeds are effective household remedy for many ailments.

Profile

Botanical Name : Coriandrum sativum

Family : Apiaceae

Appearance : Aromatic herb with dissected leaves.

Medicinal Parts : Leaves, seeds

Distribution : Coriander is native to regions spanning from southern Europe and North Africa to southwestern Asia.

Preparation and Dose

Fry in 1 tbsp ghee ½ tsp each coriander seeds, cumin seeds, black peppercorn, tail pepper and tuvar dal. Make a tasty soup by adding one tomato and 1 teacup water. Drink it as an appetizer.

7. <u>Cumin</u>

(Cuminum cyminum)

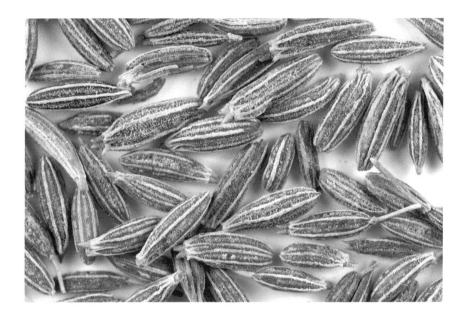

General

Cumin sometimes spelled cummin; is well known for its carminative (dispel flatus) action. It is believed that cumin has a cooling effect on the human body and hence has a definitive role in warm seasons and climates.

Profile

Botanical Name : Cuminum cyminum, Cuminum odorum

Family : Apiaceae

Appearance : A slender annual herb with angular striated stem bearing two or three partite linear blue-green leaves. Flowers – white or rose, in umbels. Fruits – grayish, about ¼ inch long, tapering towards both ends. Seeds (each one contained within a fruit, which is dried) – yellowish to grayish brown in colour.

Medicinal Parts : Fruits, often referred to as seeds

Distribution: Native from the east Mediterranean to India. Iran is major producer of cumin. Cultivated in almost all states of India except Assam region.

Prescription and Dose

Mix ½ tsp each broken cumin, coriander seeds, black peppercorn, long pepper, and tuvar dal. Boil in water. Add salt to taste. Drink it as an appetizer.

8. <u>Devil's Tree</u>

(Alstonia scholaris)

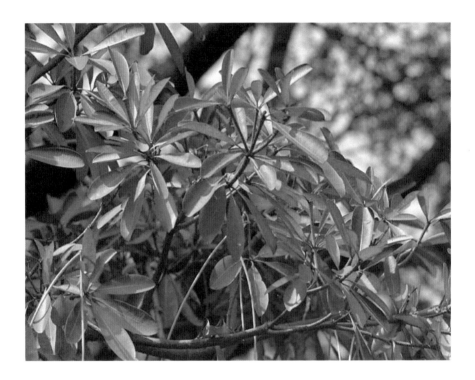

General

Commonly called Blackboard tree, Indian devil tree, Ditta bark, Milkwood pine, White cheese wood and Saptparni.

Despite its name, this tropical tree is distinguished by seven leaves in a whorl and a very bitter milky leaf juice. Its bark is pale ash-gray in colour and is commercially recognized as ditta bark.

Profile

Botanical Name : Alstonia scholaris

Family : Apocynaceae

Appearance : An ever green tree with milky juice. Bark - pale, ash gray in colour. Leaves - leathery, lance-like in whorls of 4 to7. Flowers - greenish white in terminal clusters, spice scented. Fruits - hanging in pairs, contain hairy seeds.

Medicinal Parts : Bark, milky juice, root.

Distribution : Tropical and deciduous forests of Indian subcontinent and SE Asia. It has also been naturalized in several other tropical and subtropical climates.

Prescription and Dose

Soak 3 tsp bark powder in 2 cups boiling water for 1 hour. Filter and drink 1 to 2 tbsp 2-3 tImes a day for fatigue after an illness.

9. <u>Dronapushpi</u>

(Leucas aspera)

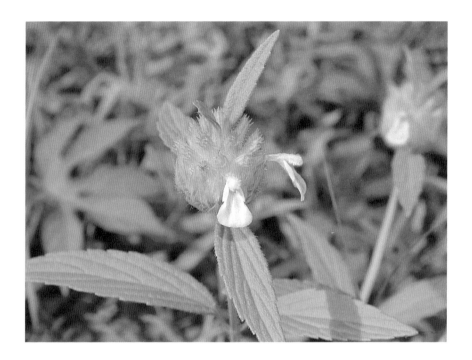

General

It has many common names, including guma, dronpushpi or drona puspi, and tou xu bai rong cao. It is a common plant across Asia from China to the Indian subcontinent.

Like many other medicinal plants, Dronapushpi grows in wilderness and in wastelands. The flowering annual herb is a common weed which also has uses as an edible vegetable and herbal remedy.

It springs up in cultivated fields as a weed, especially after a period of rain and is readily available in markets. One of the plant's most common historical uses has been as a treatment for snakebite.

Profile

Botanical Name : Leucas aspera

Other Species : Leucas cephalotes

Family : Lamiaceae

Appearance : Erect herb, 1-2 ft tall with single opposite leaves. Flowers- white, small, in axiles. Corola - 2 lipped, upper lip short and hairy, lower lip twice as long.

Medicinal Parts : Leaf, Flower

Distribution : Found in India, Bangladesh, Mauritius, and in several SE Asian countries.

Prescription and Dose

Cook a handful of leaves along with greens and a little tamarind. Eat with bread or rice during meals.

10. <u>Drumstick</u>

(Moringa oleifera)

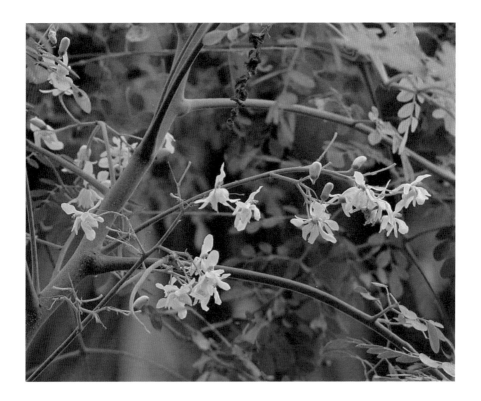

General

Because of the shape of it's fruits, the tree has come to be
called 'Drumstick'.

The fruits are rich in proteins, minerals, calcium, iron, phosphorous and vitamin C as well as facilitators such as folic acid which help in absorption of iron, and B-carotene, in synthesis of vitamin A. The creamy white flowers are also used in the treatment of several ailments. Its seeds, leaves and roots too find medicinal applications.

Profile

Botanical Name : Morianga oleifera

Family : Moringaceae

Appearance : A handsome tree with rough and cork like bark. Leaves - fern like, divided and subdivided. Flowers - while and honey scented. Fruits - elongated, 3-angular, resembling drumsticks.

Medicinal Parts : Gum, flowers, leaves, roots, seed oil

Distribution : Common throughout India.

Prescription and Dose

Boil 2 tbsp flowers in 1 cup milk. Strain and drink.

11. <u>Liquorice</u>

(Glycyrrhiza glabra)

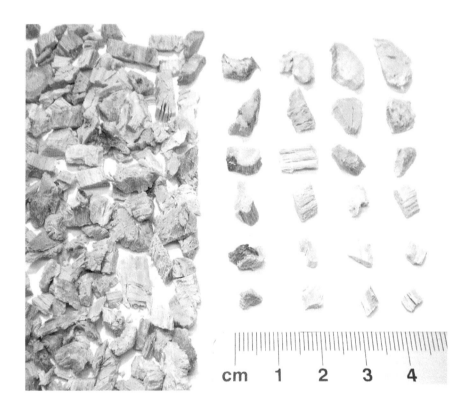

General

Liquorice or licorice is the root of Glycyrrhiza glabra from which a somewhat sweet flavor can be extracted. It has been known for thousands of years for its medicinal value. It is used to strengthen muscles and bone, curing wounds, bronchial troubles, skin diseases, ulcer and jaundice.

Profile

Botanical Name : Glycyrrhiza glabra

Family : Fabaceae

Appearance : Perennial plant found wild. The woody rootstock is wrinkled and brown on the outside, yellow inside and tastes sweet. The stem which is round on the lower part and angular higher up bears alternate odd-pinnate leaves. Leaflets are ovate and dark green in color. Flowers – yellow or purple or voilet. Pods – compressed.

Medicinal Parts : Rootstock(rhizome)

Distribution: Native to southern Europe and parts of Asia. Cultivated mostly in sub-Himalayan tracts.

Prescription and Dose

Add ¾ teacup crushed liquorice root to 4 teacups cold water and allow it to stand for 2 hours. Then bring it quickly to boil and steep for 5 minutes. Add this to bathwater in the tub.

12. Long Pepper

(Piper longum)

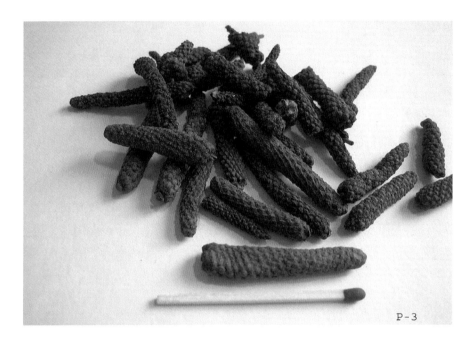

P-3

General

Long pepper, which consists of the dried fruits of the plant, is used generally as a spice. The plant is called long pepper as its spikes are longer and therefore distinguishable from black pepper. These fruits have pungent pepper like taste and produce salivation and numbness of the mouth.

Profile

Botanical Name : Piper longum

Family : Piperaceae

Appearance : Trailing or creeping aromatic plant. Leaves - dark green and shining above, but pale on lower surface. Stipules - conspicuous but soon drop off. Fruit - small, ovoid, sunk in fleshy spike. Spike - 2 to 4 cm long, oblong, blackish green, shining.

Medicinal Parts : Dried fruits, roots.

Distribution : Grows in warmer regions of India. It is readily available at Indian grocery stores.

Prescription and Dose

Mix equal quantities of the powders of long pepper and cebulik myrobalan. Add some honey. Take 1 tsp twice a day for 1-2 months.

13. <u>Mandukaparni</u>

(Centella asiatica)

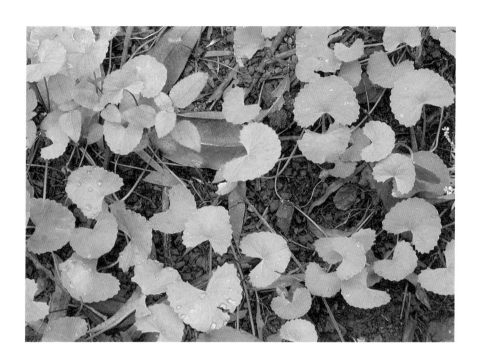

General

Mandukaparni in Sanskrit refers to shape and appearance of leaves of this plant, which resemble the webbed feet of a frog. The leaves also have a strong resemblance to human brain. The herb has been popular in the entire South East Asia besides China, Tibet, Japan and India.

Profile

Botanical Name : Centella asiatica

Other Species : Hydrocotyle asiatica

Family : Apiaceae

Appearance : A creeper bearing roots on nodes. Leaves - small, rounded/kidney shaped, with toothed margins. Flowers - pinkish red, minute, 3-6 in clusters. Fruits - small, 7-9 ridged.

Medicinal Parts : Whole plant - leaves, roots, seeds, stem

Distribution : Throughout India and SE Asia, in moist places, marshy banks of water bodies and irrigated fields.

Prescription and Dose

Pluck 10 leaves and wash in hot water. Grind them with 5 pepper corns. Mix into a glass of buttermilk and drink on an empty stomach every morning for 3 to 6 months.

For muscular fatigue, take 1/4 tsp powder of dried leaves along with honey or buttermilk.

14. <u>Mustard</u>

(Brassica nigra)

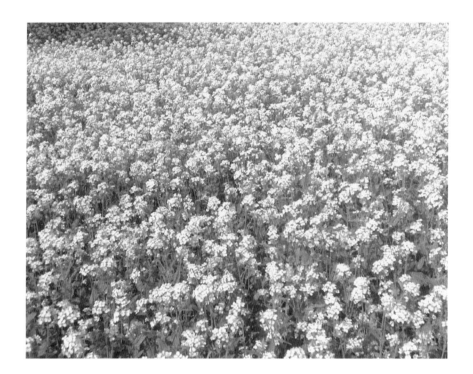

General

Mustard, which is an irritant, has also proved medicinally useful.

There are three distinct species of mustard : black, white, and brown. All three exhibit the same properties.

Profile

Botanical Name : Brassica nigra

Other Species : Brassica alba, Brassica juncea

Family : Cruciferae

Appearance : Widely cultivated annual. Leaves are alternate, lower ones bristly, upper glabrous, lance-like. Flowers are bright yellow. Black seeds develop in bulging cylindrical pods.

Medicinal Parts : Seed, oil, greens.

Distribution: White mustard grows wild in North Africa, the Middle East and Mediterranean Europe, and has spread farther; oriental mustard, originally from the foothills of the Himalaya, is grown commercially in India, Bangladesh, Canada, the UK, Denmark and the US; black mustard is grown in Argentina, Chile, the US and some European countries.

Prescription and Dose

Tie 1 teacup mustard powder in a cloth bag. Steep it for 2-3 hours in 4 teacups plain water. Remove the cloth bag and add this water to your bath water.

15. Tamarind

(Tamarindus indica)

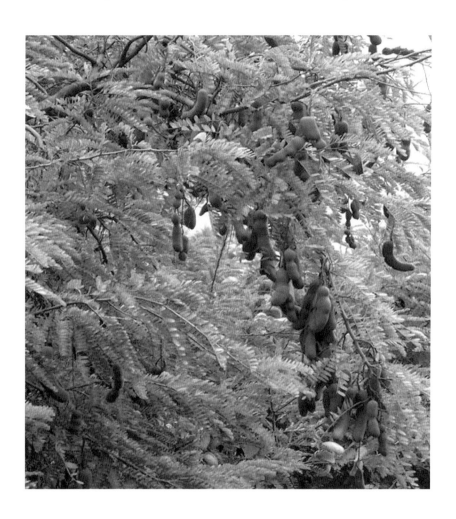

General

Tamarind is useful because of its anti-microbial and anti-bacterial properties. The tender leaves too fight worms. Apart from its use against germs, the fruit pulp also exhibits several medicinal properties - anthelmintic, carminative, digestive, laxative, and refrigerant.

It is perhaps one of the most acidic naturally occurring substances, the principal acid being tartaric acid.

Profile

Botanical Name : Tamarindus indica

Family : Leguminoseae

Appearance : A tree with small shiny leaflets. Flowers creamy yellow to pink, in clusters. Pods - thick and oblong. Seeds - brown, compressed, embedded in a fibrous, fleshy, acid pulp.

Medicinal Parts : Bark, flowers, fruits, leaves, seeds, kernel.

Distribution: Native to tropical Africa, the tree is quite common in India.

Prescription and Dose

Collect the most tender leaf buds and cook along with lentils. Temper 1/2 tsp cumin in 1 tsp ghee and add. Mix well and eat with steamed rice or bread once a day for a few weeks.

Some Important Guidelines

1. Preparation

When the herb is extremely bitter, sour, astringent or in powdered form, it can be mixed with honey, jaggery, sugar, candy etc.

2. Dosage

The quantity of dose can vary from one person to another based on individual age, physical build, and reaction of patient to a particular formulation.

The dosage prescribed in this book is meant for fully grown and mature patients. The dose should be increased/decreased for each patient keeping in mind individual patient's constitution.

3. Effectiveness

The contents of a herbal plant part varies widely due to factors such as climate, altitude, latitude, soil type, nutrition, temperature, relative humidity, time of plucking, packaging, storage etc. Hence the effectiveness of herb for treating an ailment may vary in different cases.

Patient needs to keep in mind this inherent weakness of herbal effectiveness, and be prepared to continue the treatment for a little longer time.

Other Books That May Interest You

Herbs That Cure:

Anaemia
Asthma
Bad Breath
Bleeding Piles
Constipation
Diabetes
Fatigue
Flatulence
Genito-Urinal disorders
Hair Loss
Insomnia
Joints Pain
Leucoderma
Obesity
Pimples
Psoriasis
Rheumatism
Sexual Debility
Toothache
Venereal Diseases
Wrinkles

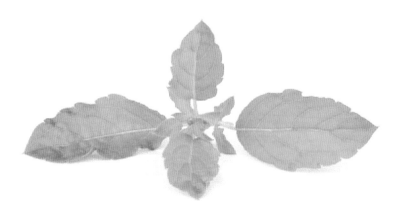

Printed in Great Britain
by Amazon